Manage Medullary Sponge Kidney:
A Patient's Guide to Managing MSK

Credits and sources are listed on final page.

ISBN: 978-1-7349073-4-6

This book was written from a patient's perspective
and is not to be used to diagnose or treat any
condition or to be used to replace medical care.

Printed in the United States of America.

Table of Contents

What is MSK?

Cacchi-Ricci Disease, primarily known as Medullary Sponge Kidney (MSK) is a congenital disorder of the kidneys. Though it is present from birth, symptoms typically do not occur until adolescence. MSK occurs when the tubules in the kidneys do not properly form in the womb. This results in cystic dilatations of the collecting tubules in one or both kidneys. On imaging scans, this shows up as a "sponge like" appearance. 70% of cases are bilateral, which means MSK occurs in both kidneys. Patients with MSK are at increased risk for kidney stones and urinary tract infection and typically pass twice as many stones per year as do other stone formers. MSK patients report chronic kidney pain, renal colic, frequent stones and recurrent infections. This kidney disease is unique because patients are, for the most part, told they are not candidates for transplant. Though MSK can cause sub-par kidney function, only 10% of patients suffer renal failure and require dialysis. If you do a google search for Medullary Sponge kidney (MSK) you will find a great deal of information that states MSK is usually a benign disorder without any symptoms, though nothing could be further from the truth.

This outdated dissonance in the medical field creates a nightmare for patients with this condition. Because medical professionals are taught that MSK is benign, patients with this condition may not receive appropriate care for their recurrent kidney stones, urinary tract infections and flank pain, especially in emergent medical settings.

This book was written from a patient's perspective who has medullary sponge kidney and also contains research and documentation that supports the truth that the condition is not always benign.

Symptoms

Commonly reported symptoms if MSK:

- Chronic kidney stone formation.
- Fatigue.
- Flank pain.
- Frequent urination.
- Hydronephrosis.
- Intolerance to dietary triggers.
- Kidney and bladder spasms.
- Pain associated with and without stone passage.

Though not present in all cases, a common marker for this disease is the formation of "Kidney Gravel." These are small, sand-like stones that some MSK patients can pass frequently. These grains cause frequent irritation in the urinary tract, which can cause pain and inflammation and can increase the risk of kidney and urinary tract infection. This "sandpaper" effect can also cause issues such as bloody urine, pain and interstitial cystitis in the bladder.

MSK is not always a benign condition, as was once thought. Patients can struggle with quality of life if the disease is not managed properly.

Diagnostics

Medullary sponge kidney is typically diagnosed with a test called an IVP (intravenous pyelogram). This procedure uses a dye contrast to allow the testing to better visualize the kidneys and expose issues such as renal duct plugging, calculi and/or cysts in the kidneys or blockages in the urinary tract. Other imaging tests can be used to evaluate diagnosed MSK for treatment protocols such as a renal ultrasound or computed tomography (CT) scan. Blood tests for calcium, phosphorus, uric acid, electrolyte levels, blood urea nitrogen (BUN), glomerular filtration rate (GFR) and creatinine levels to may also be ordered to assess kidney function. Providers should also consider running a urinalysis to check for crystals, bacteria, blood, and white cells.

24 Hour Urine Tests are also beneficial.

There are imaging tests that can determine if you have lodged or embedded stones such as: Abdominal X-ray, renal ultrasound, MRI or CT scan. It is important to note that certain types of stones may not show up on all imaging tests and if a patient is symptomatic, alternate testing is appropriate. Small stones and stones in certain locations can be more challenging to detect on imaging scans.

What causes MSK?

MSK is a congenital disorder and is present from birth. It is believed to be of genetic origin, however, there are cases where patients had no family history of MSK and other reports of families who had multiple members diagnosed with medullary sponge kidney. More research is needed to truly determine what causes this condition. MSK was previously believed not to be hereditary but there is more evidence coming forth that may indicate otherwise. There is conflicting evidence as to whether this condition is of genetic origin.

Is MSK painful?

The Journal of Nephrology published groundbreaking research[1] that validates what most Medullary Sponge Kidney patients know to be reality. Though in textbook education, doctors are taught that MSK is a benign condition that does not impact quality of life. Research is now recorded that shows MSK patients have repeated hospitalizations for stones, symptoms and pain. 71% of participants in this specific study reported daily pain that interfered strongly with everyday life and quality of life in the study, 69% of participants required pain medications daily and 70% required opioids to manage the pain associated with symptoms. The findings showed symptoms affect very negatively on the quality of life of patients diagnosed with MSK.

Survey Says

To compile accurate empirical information for this book, the following survey data reflects the personal experience of over 100 MSK patients who were anonymously surveyed.

---

[1] Gambaro, Giovanni & Goldfarb, David & Baccaro, Rocco & Hirsch, J. & Topilow, N. & D'Alonzo, S. & Gambassi, Giovanni & Ferraro, Pietro. (2018). Chronic pain in medullary sponge kidney: a rare and never described clinical presentation. Journal of Nephrology. 31. 10.1007/s40620-018-0480-8.

What age did you start having MSK symptoms?

118 responses

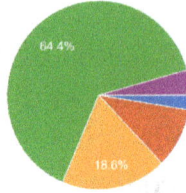

- At birth 0-1
- Early Childhood 1-12
- Teenage Years 13-19
- Early Adulthood 20-40
- Middle Age 40-60
- Older Age 60-100

64.4%

18.6%

What age were you diagnosed with MSK?

118 responses

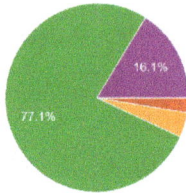

- At birth 0-1
- Early Childhood 1-12
- Teenage Years 13-19
- Early Adulthood 20-40
- Middle Age 40-60
- Older Age 60-100

16.1%

77.1%

How many kidney stones do form/get per year?

118 responses

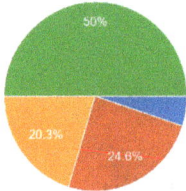

- None
- 1-5
- 5-10
- More than 10

50%

20.3%

24.6%

8

On average, do you typically pass kidney stones naturally or do you require medical intervention such as surgery, lithotripsy or ureteral stent placement?
116 responses

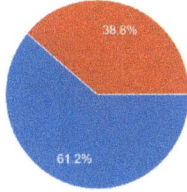

- I pass them naturally most of the time.
- I require medical intervention most of the time.

38.8%

61.2%

Have you ever had a ureteral stent?
117 responses

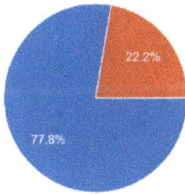

- Yes
- No

22.2%

77.8%

If so, how many ureteral stents have you had?
92 responses

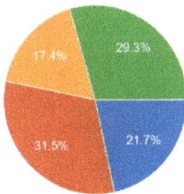

- 1
- 2-5
- 5-10
- More than 10

29.3%

17.4%

31.5%

21.7%

Have you ever had lithotripsy?
118 responses

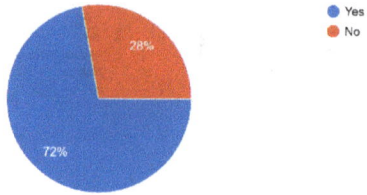

- Yes
- No

72%
28%

If so, how many lithotripsy procedures have you had?
85 responses

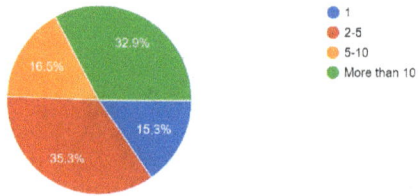

- 1
- 2-5
- 5-10
- More than 10

32.9%
16.5%
35.3%
15.3%

Have you ever passed kidney gravel? (Urinating small, sand-like kidney stone "grains")
117 responses

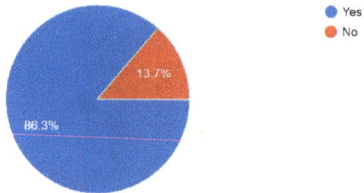

- Yes
- No

86.3%
13.7%

10

On average, how many urinary tract infections do you get per year?
118 responses

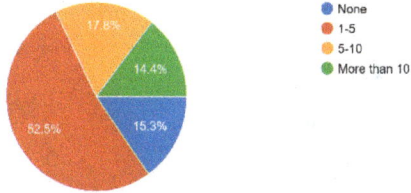

- None
- 1-5
- 5-10
- More than 10

17.8%
14.4%
52.5%
15.3%

How many times a year do you visit the emergency department for MSK related issues?
118 responses

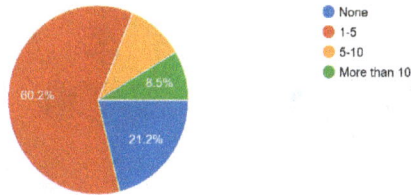

- None
- 1-5
- 5-10
- More than 10

8.5%
80.2%
21.2%

Do you have pain associated with your MSK?
117 responses

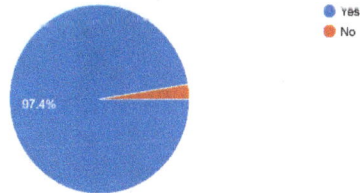

- Yes
- No

97.4%

If so, how often do you suffer with MSK related pain?

118 responses

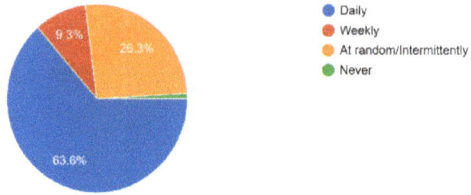

- Daily
- Weekly
- At random/Intermittently
- Never

9.3%
28.3%
63.6%

Do you suffer from kidney pain even when you are not passing a stone?

117 responses

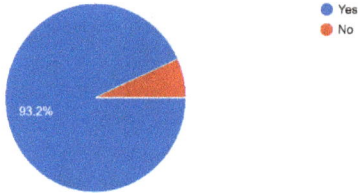

- Yes
- No

93.2%

Do you take narcotic or other pain medications for MSK related pain?

118 responses

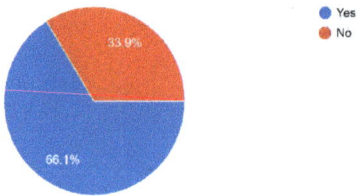

- Yes
- No

33.9%
66.1%

If so, how often do you rely on pain medication to manage MSK related pain?

104 responses

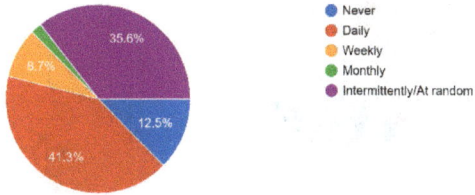

- Never
- Daily
- Weekly
- Monthly
- Intermittently/At random

35.6%
12.5%
41.3%
8.7%

Do you take any supplements or natural remedies for MSK related symptoms?

117 responses

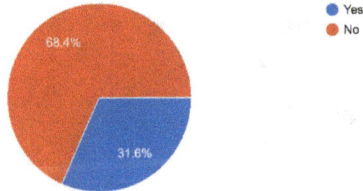

- Yes
- No

68.4%
31.6%

Do you follow a special diet to manage MSK related symptoms?

118 responses

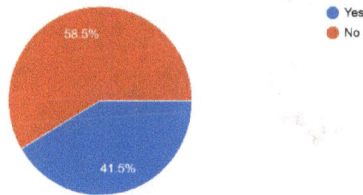

- Yes
- No

58.5%
41.5%

Do you generally feel your doctor understands how to manage your MSK?

118 responses

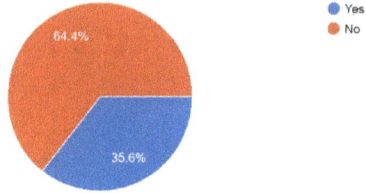

- Yes
- No

64.4%

35.6%

How many CT scans have you had specifically for MSK symptoms?

118 responses

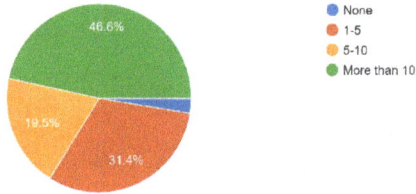

- None
- 1-5
- 5-10
- More than 10

46.6%

31.4%

19.5%

How many ultrasounds have you had specifically for MSK symptoms?

118 responses

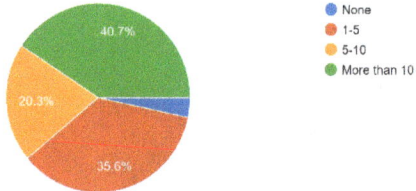

- None
- 1-5
- 5-10
- More than 10

40.7%

35.6%

20.3%

14

How many times in your life have you visited the emergency room due to MSK?

117 responses

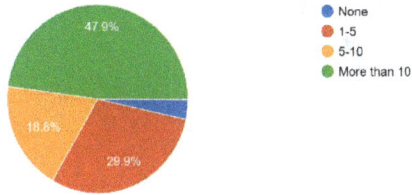

- None
- 1-5
- 5-10
- More than 10

47.9%
29.9%
18.6%

Do you feel your MSK symptoms are generally treated appropriately in an emergency care setting?

116 responses

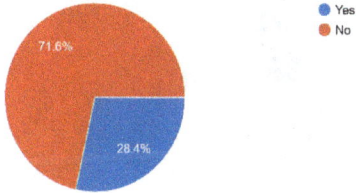

- Yes
- No

71.6%
28.4%

Have you ever been told kidney stones should not hurt because they are not "obstructive?"

117 responses

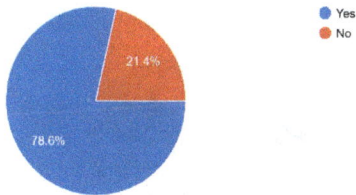

- Yes
- No

78.6%
21.4%

Do you have pain with stones even though they are not obstructive?

118 responses

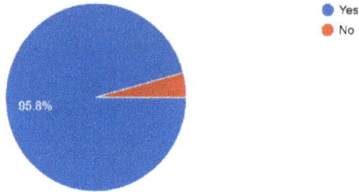

- Yes
- No

95.8%

Do you struggle with fatigue due to MSK?

118 responses

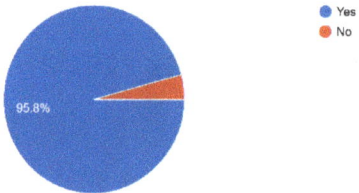

- Yes
- No

95.8%

Have MSK impacted your mental health?

117 responses

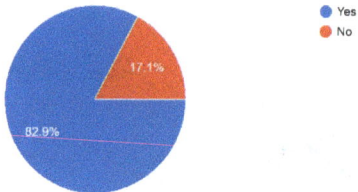

- Yes
- No

17.1%

82.9%

Would you consider your specific case of MSK to be "disabling?"
117 responses

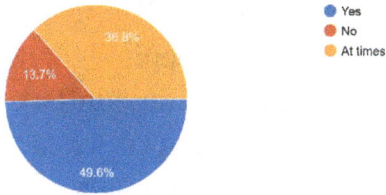

- Yes
- No
- At times

36.8%
13.7%
49.6%

Have you tried any alternative therapies to manage your MSK?
118 responses

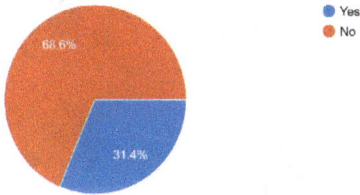

- Yes
- No

68.6%
31.4%

Do you have any other health conditions other than MSK?
117 responses

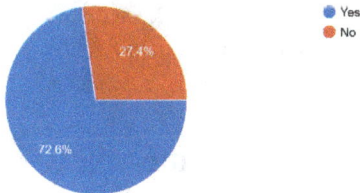

- Yes
- No

27.4%
72.6%

As you can see from the survey results, medullary sponge kidney is far from a "benign condition" and carries with it a myriad of challenges. In addition to the misnomer that it is a benign condition, doctors need to be aware that medullary sponge kidney can also cause pain, even when not associated with active stone passage. Renal colic, flank pain and fatigue are commonly reported by patients, even when not passing an active stone. Stone pain is also reported when stones are in the kidney. Nonobstructive stones can cause pain.

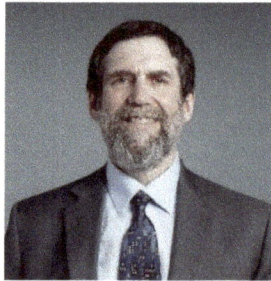

The following letter was written by one of the leading experts on Medullary Sponge Kidney, Dr. David S. Goldfarb. He is the Clinical Chief of Nephrology at NY Harbor VA Medical Center-NYU Langone Hospital. His practice provides care to one of the largest MSK populations in the United States and he has written several scientific articles about the condition.

NYU School of Medicine

NYU LANGONE MEDICAL CENTER

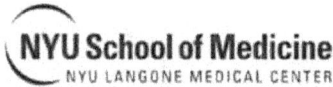

David S. Goldfarb, M.D.
Clinical Chief, Division of Nephrology
New York University Medical Center
Professor of Medicine and Physiology
NYU School of Medicine

Nephrology Section, NYVAMC
423 E. 23rd St., New York, NY 10010
Telephone: (212) 263-0744
Facsimile: (212) 951-6842
Email: david.goldfarb@nyumc.org

February 13, 2014

Re: Medullary sponge kidney

Dear Healthcare Professional,

Medullary sponge kidney (MSK) is a relatively rare disorder of the kidneys which leads to frequent kidney stones. People with MSK often tend to have significantly worse than run-of-the-mill kidney stone disease.

I have one of the largest MSK populations in the United States and I have written several scientific articles about this disorder. The disease is extremely variable and affects quality of life in a way that can be quite difficult. It may be difficult to manage even with the best intentions and adherence to prescriptions.

Many patients have recurrent stones and require visits to Emergency Rooms. The diagnosis of renal colic in a patient with MSK is usually obvious. Failure of stone passage despite NSAIDs and tamsulosin might warrant an ultrasound. CT scans can be reserved for more persistent renal colic as the relatively young average age of onset leads to excessive radiation exposure over the course of a lifetime.

The most important means of prevention of stones is drinking lots of fluids. The result is the need to urinate frequently as well. People with MSK should be permitted to have liquids with them at all times and have liberal bathroom privileges as well.

Pain medications are often necessary on a chronic basis. While physicians usually claim that patients who do not have obstructing stones on imaging do not experience pain, this has not been supported by my clinical practice. Many patients have chronic pain syndromes that require chronic use of NSAIDs, opiates such as Percocet and Vicodin or methadone. Many patients with these chronic pain syndromes are able to attend school and work if properly medicated. On the other hand, disability may result and some people simply cannot work or attend school for longer periods of time.

I am happy to help take care of patients with MSK at a distance. If you have questions or comments regarding the management of affected people, you are welcome to email or call me any time. I appreciate your empathetic care of this deserving group of beleaguered patients.

Yours truly,

David S. Goldfarb, M.D.
Clinical Chief, Nephrology Division,
NYU Medical Center
Professor of Medicine and Physiology,
NYU School of Medicine

19

His letter reads:

Dear Healthcare Professional,

Medullary Sponge Kidney (MSK) is a relatively rare disorder of the kidneys which leads to frequent kidney stones. People with MSK often tend to have a significantly worse than run-of-the-mill kidney stone disease. I have one of the largest MSK populations in the United States and have written several scientific articles about this disorder. This disease is extremely variable and affects quality of life in a way that can be quite difficult. It may be difficult to manage even with the best intentions and adherence to prescriptions. Many patients have recurrent stones that require visits to emergency rooms. The diagnosis of renal colic in a patient with MSK is usually obvious. The failure of stone passage despite NSAIDs and tamsulosin might warrant an ultrasound. CT scans can be reserved for more persistent renal colic as the relatively young average of age of onset leads to excessive radiation exposure over the course of a lifetime. The most important means of prevention of stones is drinking lots of fluid. The result is the need to urinate frequently as well. People with MSK should be permitted to have liquids with them at all times and have liberal bathroom privileges as well. Pain medications are often necessary on a chronic basis. While physicians usually claim that patients who do not have obstructing stones on imaging do not experience pain, this has not been supported by my clinical practice. Many patients who have chronic pain syndromes that require chronic use of NSAIDs and opioids such as Percocet or Vicodin or methadone. Many patients with these chronic pain syndromes are able to attend school and work if properly medicated. On the other hand, disability may result and some people simply cannot work or attend school for long periods of time. I am happy to take care of patients with MSK at a distance. If you have questions or comments regarding the management of affected people, you are welcome to e-mail or call me at any time period. I appreciate your empathetic care of this deserving group of beleaguered patients.

Yours truly,

David S. Goldfarb
Clinical Chief, Nephrology Division- NYU Medical Center
Professor of Medicine and Physiology
NYU School of Medicine

As acknowledged in Dr. Goldfarb's letter, Medullary Sponge Kidney can be a difficult condition to manage and sometimes pain medication is necessary to achieve quality of life.

Doctors should try to treat the source of pain instead of masking it with medication, but the truth is, sometimes narcotic medications are necessary for quality of life. When managing debilitating conditions, the denial of properly prescribed, safely used medications to treat incurable, chronic pain is inhumane. Properly used opioids are used to give quality of life to those suffering with incurable, chronic pain. If you have chronic pain, don't suffer needlessly. There is no shame in becoming a pain clinic patient. This does not mean you are an addict. This just means you need help managing a painful condition. If you have unmanaged pain, please contact a physician. Don't lose hope, narcotics are not your only option. There are many modalities that can aid in the fight against kidney pain and stone formation.

Medications for MSK

(Do not start or stop any medications, supplements, or treatments without first consulting your physician. This information is only to be used as a patient's perspective and not to be used to treat or diagnose any condition. Contact your

doctor regarding the use of any medications or treatments.)

Ditropan (generic name- oxybutynin)- Antispasmodic and anticholinergic medication used to treat symptoms of overactive bladder but also found to be beneficial in patients with renal colic.

Levsin (generic name- hyoscyamine)- Antispasmodic medication beneficial in quelling renal colic and bladder spasms.

Atarax (generic name- hydroxyzine)- Antihistamine medication used to reduce pain and inflammation.

Elavil (generic-amitriptyline)- Tricyclic antidepressant medication used to reduce pain and may also help those suffering from depression due to chronic pain.

Elmiron (generic name- pentosan polysulfate sodium)- Mildly blood thinning medication that also works as a bladder protectant and is prescribed to treat bladder pain and discomfort.

Flomax (generic name- tamsulosin hydrochloride)- Alpha-blocker medication that relaxes the urinary tract, making it easier to urinate and pass stones. *(Be careful if you have a sulfa allergy if considering this medication.)*

Utira-C Tablets (generic name- hyoscyamine, methenamine, methylene blue, phenyl salicylate, sodium biphosphate)-Prescription medicine that contains multiple medications used in combination to treat urinary pain, spasms and inflammation.

Pyridium (generic name-phenazopyridine)- Analgesic medication used for relief of pain, burning and urgency of the lower urinary tract.

Alternative Options

(Disclaimer- This is not a complete list of all possible non-medicinal options. For more information, please consult your physician or holistic health practitioner.)

Acupuncture- To explain acupuncture in a western medical way, acupuncture needles stimulate the central nervous system, which in turn, stimulates the body's natural healing abilities to promote physical and emotional well-being. Acupuncture also helps the body to release natural endorphins, which can aid in pain relief and stress reduction.

Bladder instillations- These treatments may be beneficial if your MSK causes you to have interstitial cystitis symptoms. These treatments are performed by inserting a catheter into the bladder and filling it with a combination of medications to treat the symptoms of burning pain or interstitial cystitis. The combination is inserted into the bladder and the patient "holds" the liquids for as long as possible. The medications reduce inflammation and discomfort within the bladder. A urologist can prescribe this treatment and it is an outpatient procedure, usually performed by a nurse.

Frequency Therapy- Frequency therapy is a non-invasive, non-medicinal alternative treatment. It is highly personalized because protocols are adapted to the patient's specific needs. Thousands of protocols offer options for a wide variety of symptoms both physical and emotional which may have been otherwise deemed "untreatable." Since it has such a high success rate, top medical systems such as Cleveland Clinic are now offering frequency therapy as a treatment option.
Frequency therapy is used to help the body enter a natural healing state. Precise frequencies can target harmful substances at the source and accelerate the body's natural recovery at the cellular level. Frequency devices use soundwaves and microcurrents that are programmed to impact certain parts of the body through "protocols." These machines have many protocols for pain, injury and relaxation. The frequencies used during

treatment are extremely mild, one millionth of an ampere. Such a small amount of electrical current is safe because the human body naturally produces its own current within each of your cells.

Patient's Perspective Note- I was introduced to frequency microcurrent treatment before I got a formal diagnosis of Medullary Sponge kidney. One of the physicians over my care was an integrative doctor who used natural remedies in addition to western medical care. He convinced me to use the frequency machine to help manage my renal colic and pain. To my surprise, the machine decreased my pain levels. The treatment was so beneficial that I ended up getting the training and purchasing a machine myself. I now not only use frequency medicine personally, but also use it in my holistic practice to help my patients.

Heating Pad- Heating pads can be your best friend if you struggle with MSK pain. Be sure to never fall asleep on it and always be vigilant of the heat settings to prevent burns. Use extra caution if you are diabetic or on blood thinning medication.

Pelvic Floor Therapy- Passing chronic kidney stones can cause a lot of physical problems. Chronic urinary tract pain can lead to other issues such as voiding dysfunction and interstitial cystitis. PVT can help treat these issues. People with chronic kidney stones are also prone to develop chronic back pain due to the tendency to "tense" up from the pain of stones. Physical therapy can help you relax those tense muscles and help eliminate trigger points and spasms. Most insurance will cover this if your doctor refers you.

Aqua Therapy- Exercising with chronic pain can feel like an impossible task. Water therapy is a great way to exercise in a way that causes less pressure on your joints, muscles and frankly your whole body. Movement has been researched to help stone passage. This is a great way to get moving in a gentle, low impact environment.

TENS Unit- (Transcutaneous electrical nerve stimulation) A machine that uses electrical current pulses produced by a device to stimulate the nerves for pain relief. To use, you simply place the electrode pads on the affected area and turn the frequency to a comfortable pulse. It is believed to help release the tension caused by chronic pain by calming the nerve impulses.

Herbalism- Herbal medicine has been used since the dawn of time to help reduce pain and manage symptoms of all sorts of conditions. Herbal medicine, however, needs to be administered safely and effectively. Just because something is natural does not mean it is safe. Herbs can interact with certain medications, so be sure to get advice from a clinical herbalist before you start any herb. You can also consult your doctor as well but be warned that they are not always trained in herbal medicine. Though you should not diagnose or treat yourself, you can always go into medical journals and research websites such as PubMed to find scientific research on herbal medicine.

Patient Perspective Note- As a clinical herbalist who also suffers from MSK, I use many herbal remedies to manage my symptoms. They are not cures, but they can help manage pain, nausea and discomfort.

Essential Oils- There are various essential oils used for various things such as pain management and relaxation. There are many holistic practitioners and aromatherapists that can help you discover which EO's are right for you. These modalities are not cures for MSK, but they can be beneficial in improving your quality of life.

Supplements

(Disclaimer- This is not a complete list of all possible natural supplements. Do not start any supplement without first checking with both a healthcare provider and clinical herbalist.)

IP-6 Inositol- A vitamin-like substance found in seeds that has been reported to prevent the formation of kidney stones. It is also used as an immune support and cancer fighter.

Chanca Piedra- An herb believed to relieved to aid in dissolving kidney stones, increase urine output and have activity against bacteria and viruses, also believed to help lower blood sugar. (Diabetics and people with hypoglycemia should use this with caution.)

Oregano Oil or Capsules- Oregano is a natural antimicrobial and can be used to prevent infection caused by kidney stones.

Uva Ursi (Bearberry)- Uva ursi, also known as bearberry, has been used medicinally by Native Americans for centuries. It was commonly used as a treatment for bladder-related infections before the discovery of sulfa drugs and antibiotics.

Horsetail- Horsetail is one of the first line herbal remedies for kidney stones because of its diuretic properties which increase urine output and can reduce renal colic. However, horsetail may flush potassium out of the body so people who are at risk for low potassium levels should not take it.

Marshmallow Root- Natural herbal anti-inflammatory used to lessen the inflammation in the urinary and respiratory tracts. Can be ingested in the form of capsules, powder or made into a warm tea.

Health Care with MSK

Find a Good Doctor

Finding a good doctor willing to help you is essential in managing medullary sponge kidney. You deserve to find the right doctor who will not only treat your symptoms but validate you as a patient. There are countless urologists and nephrologists practicing medicine. You can find one that is willing to help you manage your health issues. Don't be afraid to "fire" a doctor that isn't helping you. This is your life, your body and your disease. You deserve to find answers. Don't give up until you find the proper care you deserve.

You can also reach out to online support groups for referrals. Social media can be a great resource to find people who may share your condition or symptoms. You can connect with people all across the world who may share in your hardships. Other patients may help direct you to the right doctor. A word of caution, however, is not to use the internet to replace medical advice and to disengage if support groups become a source of stress. Social media can be a great resource; just be sure you are selective in who you interact with and never replace your medical care with social media suggestions.

It is also important to "Do your homework." Be sure to have personal copies of your medical record or access to them in a patient portal to send them to the doctor before your appointment. This will give the physician a chance to understand your case and form a plan of action for treatment.

According to the National Institutes of Health research[2], doctors only spend an average of fifteen minutes with each patient. It is difficult to explain your entire health history and form a proper treatment plan in such a short time period. Giving your doctor a "heads up" will give them a chance to fully understand your case. This will give you the best chance of managing your illness. When the doctor has a full understanding, they can better formulate a plan for you.

---

[2] Tai-Seale, Ming et al. "Time allocation in primary care office visits." Health services research vol. 42,5 (2007): 1871-94. doi:10.1111/j.1475-6773.2006.00689.x

It is your responsibility to advocate for yourself and voice your concerns. If you are in pain, be honest about it. If you are constantly passing stones, let your doctor know. If you are struggling, don't suffer in silence. Don't be afraid to tell the truth. A good doctor will want to help you and not label you as a drug seeker.

It is also vital to keep a health log. Keep a daily journal of your symptoms, the foods and beverages you ingest, the stressors in your life and the amount of sleep you're getting.

Getting a full picture of your own health can help your doctor manage your symptoms and show you when you need to eliminate things such as dietary or environmental triggers.

Determine your type of Kidney Stones

(Disclaimer- These are basic explanations of the most commonly formed kidney stones. For a complete list of kidney stone types, please consult your urologist for more information.)

Calcium oxalate- The most common form of kidney stones, usually in the form of calcium oxalate. Oxalate is a naturally occurring substance found in certain foods and is also made by your liver.

Calcium phosphate- This type of stone is more common in patients with chronic metabolic conditions such as renal tubular acidosis (condition where the kidneys fail to properly acidify urine) hyperparathyroidism (when the body produces too much parathyroid hormone) and urinary tract infections.

Struvite- Struvite, also known as staghorn stones, form due to urinary tract or kidney infections.

Uric acid- Uric acid stones typically form in patients who are dehydrated and are more prevalent in people who eat a high-protein diet. People with gout also have increased risk of creating this type of stone. Genetic factors also may increase the risk of uric acid stones.

Cystine- This type of stone is found in people with a hereditary disorder that causes the kidneys to excrete too much of certain amino acids (cystinuria).

Testing & Evaluation of Stone Factors

If you collect a stone that you've passed, your doctor can issue a lab order to have it analyzed. This will tell you what your stones are made of and help you figure out the source. It is imperative you know what type of stone your body creates. You cannot battle something you don't fully understand. It is also vital to examine what factors can impact your stone formation. Everyone is different and may not have the same triggers. People with genetic factors may have a harder time managing kidney stones because they are not always caused by an external problem such as dehydration.

Emergency Room Visits

Visiting the emergency room can be a very daunting process. It is often packed with irritable people who are in pain, sick and impatient. Making the decision to go the emergency room is something that chronic pain patients often ponder.

"Do I need to go to the emergency room, or should I just suffer at home?"

This question is one only you can answer, but as a word of caution, keep in mind the emergency room's primary role in medicine is to handle traumatic situations such as car wrecks, heart attacks and broken bones. It is for the treatment of acute situations and not a place for extensive diagnostics. The doctors, nurses and care staff are trained to handle acute situations. Which is not to say diagnostics do not happen in the emergency department, but for the most part the staff is trained to quickly assess, treat and clear the room for the next acute situation. The emergency room is great for acute situations, but they may not have the staffing or resources in their department to figure out anyone's extensive health puzzle. Their objectives are to stabilize a patient, make sure they are not in a critical, life-threatening state and discharge them.

Kidney stones are a horrific, painful experience. They are one of the top ten reasons people visit the emergency room. Kidney stones become life threatening when they become obstructed. The emergency department staff are trained to handle life threatening situations quickly, but pain management is not the main concern of emergency room staff. This is why finding a good urologist or nephrologist is essential to treating your kidney issues. They can spend time with you at your appointments and are not in a rush to clear a bed for an acute patient. These doctors can run extensive diagnostic tests to help discover how to better help you.

In the emergency room setting, the first line kidney stone treatment protocol is typically to push fluids and manage pain. The emergency department may or may not give you pain medication or administer IV fluids for your kidney stones. This choice depends on the physician treating you. Some are more compassionate than others, as some believe kidney stones only hurt when they are moving or obstructive. You know your body, if you feel that you need medical intervention, please don't hesitate to visit the emergency room.

Knowing the following information may help you in deciding whether to go to the emergency room for your kidney stone.

- Ability to urinate.
- Blood pressure.
- Heart rate.
- Oxygen saturation.
- Pain levels.
- Respirations.
- Temperature.

Surgical Interventions

(Disclaimer- This is not a complete list of all possible surgical options. For more information, please consult your physician.)

Shockwave Lithotripsy- A common procedure performed under general anesthesia where sound waves are focused on renal calculi, resulting in the breaking of the stone(s) into small fragments. The stone fragments are then excreted through the urine.

Cystoscopy- A procedure where your doctor examines the lining of your bladder and urethra by using a hollow tube called a cystoscope. This tube is inserted into your bladder and can be used to diagnose bladder issues such as interstitial cystitis, tissue damage or stones in the bladder.

Ureteroscopy- A procedure where a scope is inserted through the urethra, bladder and into the kidney for removal of ureteral stones. The surgeon grabs the stone and removes it from the kidney or ureter. This is typically an outpatient procedure.

Percutaneous Nephrolithotomy- A procedure where the surgeon makes a small incision in the back, then by using a nephroscope (a miniature fiberoptic camera) removes the stone.

Kidney Stents

If you have been diagnosed with Medullary Sponge Kidney, odds are you will have a conversation about kidney stents at some point with your healthcare provider. This chapter will discuss everything you need to know about these "necessary evils."

What are Kidney Stents?

Kidney stents, also called ureteral stents, are tubes that allow urine to flow from the kidneys into the bladder. They are placed to prevent ureteral obstructions from kidney stones and used to treat issues such as hydronephrosis, which is a condition where the kidneys swell due to excess fluid. Stents are usually temporary, but people with chronic kidney problems may need ureteral stents replaced every few months. On average, ureteral stents are about 10 to 15 inches long and about ¼ inch in diameter. They line the entire length of the ureter to keep it open. The top part of the stent has a coil that sits inside the kidney and there is a loop at the lower end which sits inside the bladder.

Are Stents Painful?

Kidney stents are unfortunately painful, but no more so than having hydronephrosis or passing a kidney stone. Most MSK patients do find they get relief after they have been successfully treated with stents. Patients typically require the use of pain-relieving medications while the stents are in their body, especially immediately after insertion.

Other medications used to help manage comfort with stents are urinary medications such as Ditropan, myrbetriq, uribel, utira-c or levsin.

Bladder irritation and urinary frequency are common, in addition to the sensation of incomplete voiding. Stent pain is typically reported as discomfort and a dull ache in the groin or lower back pain. It can occasionally be sharp and may increase with physical activity or sitting/sleeping in a position which causes increased pressure to the area. These symptoms should subside once the stent has been removed.

How are they inserted?

This procedure is typically done under general anesthesia. The surgeon will insert a small scope device called a cystoscope through the urethra and into the bladder, then threads a flexible wire through the cystoscope into the ureter and places the ureteral stent. The curled part of the stent sits in the kidney, while another curled part rests in the bladder. Lastly, the surgeon removes the guidewire and cystoscope, leaving the stent in place.

How are they removed?

Though the stents are typically placed under general anesthesia, they are usually removed in the doctor's office without sedation. This sounds like a terrifying experience but is far less painful than a kidney stone.

To remove the stent, the doctor inserts a cystoscope through the urethra and into the bladder and inserts tiny clamps attached to the cystoscope to remove the stent out of your body.

Before your stent removal, take your prescribed pain medications, hydrate and relax. The procedure only takes a few minutes and is tolerable. It sounds far worse than it actually is. The pain of stent removal is nowhere near the pain of a kidney stone. Take heart that stent removal is nothing to be afraid of and is over in mere moments.

Some short-term ureteral stents have strings that hang outside the urethra, your healthcare provider may instruct you to gently pull on the string to remove it yourself.

Frequently Asked Questions

Can I drive with a stent?

If you are on narcotic medications to manage the pain of a stent, no. However, if you are not taking medications which inhibit your ability to drive, you can do so a few days after your procedure. It is important to allow your body to adjust after you have received anesthesia, so as a general rule of caution, it is recommended to wait at least a week to resume normal driving activity.

Is sexual activity safe with a stent?

Having an indwelling kidney stent is not the most comfortable experience, so sexual activity may not even be a concern or desire. If there is no string attached to the stent, there are no restrictions on sexual activity. However, sex can exacerbate stent discomfort, cause pain, increase blood in your urine and may not be an enjoyable experience.

If your doctor placed a string attached to your stent, do not have sexual activity. The stent may get dislodged and cause injury to the urethra. Sexual contact can also increase infection risk, so it may be best to restrict sexual activity until after your stent is removed.

Should I avoid exercise?

It is common to have blood in the urine immediately after stent placement. Activity can also exacerbate discomfort and blood in the urine, so it is best to restrict strenuous activity while you have kidney stents in place. Consider abstaining from activities that cause your urine to become bloody or causes pain that is not controlled with medication.

How do I sleep with a stent?

Sleep is vital when you're recovering from a ureteral stent placement. Your body needs rest to heal, but it can be difficult to find a comfortable position with stents. One option is to ask your doctor to prescribe medications to reduce renal spasms and urinary discomfort such as: ditropan, myrbetriq, uribel, utira-c or levsin. You can also try some holistic remedies to help you rest such as drinking chamomile or passionflower tea to help you relax and fall asleep. Taking a hot bath before bed may also help soothe the discomfort and induce sleep. There is no established "best" position for reducing stent-related discomfort when sleeping, however, some people feel better sleeping on the opposite side where their stent is placed, but that is less than helpful if you have bilateral stents. Kidney stents are uncomfortable yet can be a necessary intervention for medullary sponge kidney management. If you experience discomfort that is uncontrolled, please contact your doctor immediately.

Urinary Tract Infections (UTI)

Patients who struggle with kidney stones are at increased risk of developing urinary tract infections. If you are a chronic UTI sufferer, it is imperative you get frequent urinalysis testing with your physician to prevent sepsis. If you suspect you have a UTI, call your doctor as soon as possible.

Possible Symptoms of UTI

- Bladder pain (cystitis)
- Blood in urine.
- Burning with urination.
- Fever.
- Frequent urges to urinate.

- Lower abdominal discomfort.
- Nausea.
- Painful urination.
- Pelvic pressure.
- Shaking and/or chills.
- Vomiting.

Patients who struggle with kidney stones are at increased risk of developing urinary tract infections. Chronic UTI sufferers should get routine urinalysis testing completed. At home test strips can be beneficial to assessing whether infection is present, however at home tests may not be as accurate as laboratory testing, so it is important to communicate with your healthcare provider if you are exhibiting symptoms. Everyone is unique and can experience different symptoms.

UTI Prevention

(The following suggestions are from a patient's perspective and are not to be used to replace medical care. Do not start any medications, treatments, diets, or therapies without first consulting your healthcare provider.)

In chronic stone formers, the chance for contracting urinary tract infections is increased.

However, there are many proactive steps you can take to prevent UTI's.

Hydration- This is the first defense in preventing urinary tract infections. When you are dehydrated, your body does not have the proper fluid content to perform at optimal function. Dehydration can also lead to the formation of kidney stones. Do yourself a favor and drink an adequate amount of water every single day.

Oregano Oil or Capsules- Oregano contains active biological substances which researchers have discovered it has the ability to stop bacteria from producing urease (a substance found in pathogenic bacteria.) Many studies have shown that oregano has some of the strongest urease-inhibiting phenols. Some patients have found when ingesting oregano oil or capsules they see a decrease in urinary tract infections.

D-mannose- A simple sugar derived from fruits and is naturally found in certain cells in the human body. This powder or supplement is used for preventing urinary tract infections. It works by inhibiting bacteria from bonding to the urinary tract, therefore preventing infections.

Topical Probiotic Spray- Topical probiotics have good bacteria that work as microscopic cleaners that break up biofilm by killing the harmful bacteria and leaving the good bacteria to thrive. Especially beneficial for use after intimate contact /sexual activity. To use, apply 1-2 sprays on genital area after bathing and sexual activity.

Patient Perspective Note- I have found great success with the topical probiotic spray brand, Siani Probiotic Care. You can find their product at- probioticbodycare.com

Lifestyle UTI Prevention Tips

- Urinate as you feel the need to.
- Use natural, unscented feminine products.
- Use quality toilet paper and wipe properly after using the restroom.
- Urinate after intimate contact/sexual activity and bathe afterwards.
- Wear comfortable cotton undergarments in your proper size and change them daily.
- Avoid staying in wet clothing such as bathing suits/swim trunks.
- Practice proper hygiene and perineal care.
- Take all your medications as prescribed.
- Avoid excess sugar and eat nutritiously.

Treatment Concerns

Antibiotics are beneficial in the management of urinary tract infections but can also cause secondary issues such as candida, C-diff infections and antibiotic resistance.

Candida- An overgrowth of fungus that occurs when the PH balance in the body is disrupted and can be caused by antibiotic, oral contraceptive, or corticosteroid use. Using probiotics in addition to your antibiotics may prevent you from developing candida.

Possible Symptoms of Candida

(Disclaimer- This is not a complete list of all possible symptoms, for more information please consult your physician.)

- Allergies
- Bad breath.
- Bloating.
- Exhaustion.
- Hormonal imbalance.
- Joint pain.
- Low libido.
- Sugar cravings.
- Weakened immune system.
- White coating on tongue.

The treatment for candida is typically oral anti-fungal medications, probiotics and eliminating sugar from your diet. If you suspect you are suffering from candida, contact your healthcare provider.

Clostridium difficile (C-diff)- Occurs when the healthy bacteria in the colon is disrupted, often from the use of antibiotics. Though the C. diff bacteria is commonly found in soil, water, and feces, it is a contagious infection and can cause colon damage.

Possible Symptoms of C-Diff

- Abdominal cramping.
- Dehydration.
- Diarrhea.
- Fever.
- Loss of appetite.
- Nausea.
- Rapid heart rate.
- Weight loss.

If you are having any of these symptoms, consult your doctor. They can order diagnostic tests to determine if you have an active C-diff infection. You will have to provide a stool sample for testing and your doctor can determine if you need further treatment. The treatment of C-diff are medications such as metronidazole, vancomycin fidaxomicin which are commonly used in the management of this issue. In extreme cases, surgical interventions are also used if colon damage has occurred.

Sepsis

When infections, bacteria or germs enter a human body and are not properly treated it can cause sepsis. Septic shock has a fifty percent mortality rate, which is why urinary tract infections must be addressed with timely and appropriate treatment.

Possible Symptoms of Sepsis

- Breathing rate higher than 20 breaths per minute.
- Clammy, sweaty skin.
- Confusion or disorientation.
- Extreme pain or discomfort.
- High heart rate.
- Probable or confirmed infection.
- Shivering or feeling very cold.
- Shortness of breath.
- Temperature changes such as fever at or above 100°F or a temperature below 96.8°F.
- Unconsciousness.
- Weakness.

If you suspect you have a severe infection or could be septic, visit your local emergency room immediately. Sepsis can turn deadly extremely quickly. Therefore, it is imperative to have frequent urinalysis testing if you are a chronic stone former.

Antibiotics

Antibiotic resistance- The process of bacteria mutating to the point it inhibits the effectiveness of medications used to treat infections; therefore, causing the antibiotics to be ineffective in curing infections.

Antibiotics are typically the first line treatment in managing urinary tract infections. It is important to completely finish your antibiotic treatment to completely eradicate the infection.

Antibiotic resistance can occur if you abruptly stop treatment before the full course of antibiotics have been administered.

Diet and MSK

Most patients require a combination of dietary and lifestyle changes to manage medullary sponge kidney. Properly formulating a dietary plan involves the following steps:

1.Understand what types of stones your body makes.

This will help determine what foods you may need to avoid. You can accomplish this by having stones you have passed tested in a laboratory to discover their content and also by completing a 24-hour urine testing panel by a company such as Litholink.

2.Keep a daily log of your diet, hydration and symptoms.

You need to know what foods you are eating to determine if those foods are causing symptoms. You also need to keep track of your water intake to evaluate how well your body can hydrate itself.

3. Create a "Game Plan" Based on the above information, you will need to create a diet protocol that is actionable. If you create meal plans full of foods you do not like or cannot successfully sustain, your diet will not be successful.

Low Oxalate Diet

Many MSK patients have found great success with a low oxalate diet protocol. Oxalates, also known as oxalic acid, are naturally occurring compounds in certain foods. When eaten, oxalates bind to minerals and compounds such as calcium oxalate and iron oxalate. Oxalate diets have been linked to an increased risk of kidney stones, which is why it can be an optimal choice for sufferers of MSK. Though it may not fully stop stone formation, it has been shown to decrease the size and frequency of stones, thus reducing the frequency of kidney stents and other renal emergencies in some patients.

On a low oxalate diet, the limit for daily oxalate to 40 to 50mg. Vitamin C can also be converted into oxalate when it's metabolized. Patients following a low oxalate protocol are advised to avoid high amounts of Vitamin C and eat only low oxalate foods.

This diet protocol is surprising because most high oxalate foods are considered to be "healthy." Many MSK patients find the foods they were eating to improve their health were in fact, increasing their stone formation. For example, carrots, celery, and beets are touted as "superfoods." Many chronic stone formers are encouraged to drink daily celery juice to help them "detox" and "flush" their kidneys, while unknowingly creating a toxic buildup of oxalic acid in their body. Another "healthy" replacement that can wreak havoc on MSK symptoms is almond milk. Dairy products are denounced by many health professionals and said to be inflammatory, but the calcium in dairy products can actually help bind oxalates. Dietary calcium binds to oxalate before it gets to the kidneys, there helping to prevent stone formation. Almond milk, however, is extremely high in oxalate and can increase the prevalence of kidney stones. Pairing high oxalate foods with calcium-rich foods helps to dilute oxalates. However, on this diet, it is best to avoid high oxalate foods and keep your max oxalate intake lower than 50mg per day.

Arguably, the best resource available on the low oxalate diet protocol is the work done by Sally K. Norton. Her book, <u>Toxic Superfoods: How Oxalate Overload Is Making You Sick--and How to Get Better</u> is an invaluable resource for those pursuing a low oxalate lifestyle. Information on her research is available for free on her website: **sallyknorton.com**.

I also have social media accounts: Facebook.com/lowoxalatelifestyle and @lowoxalatelifestyle on Instagram where I share free recipes and resources for low oxalate life.

Hydronephrosis

Hydronephrosis is a condition caused by excess fluid in one or both kidneys due to a backup of urine. The most common symptom of this condition is flank pain, but other symptoms can include pain during urination, increased urge or frequency, incomplete urination, incontinence, nausea and fever. These symptoms depend on the cause and severity. Medullary sponge kidney can be a direct cause of hydronephrosis due to the impact of the small cysts that form either on tiny tubes within the kidney or the collecting ducts.

These cysts can reduce the outward flow of urine from the kidneys[3].

How is Hydronephrosis Diagnosed?

Renal ultrasound is typically used to confirm a diagnosis. CT scans can also be used to diagnose this condition, however in MSK patients, the frequent need for imaging usually warrants the use of imaging with less radiation exposure such as ultrasound. Urinalysis testing can also be ordered to evaluate if infection is the source of the hydronephrosis.

How is Hydronephrosis Treated?

The treatment for hydronephrosis is dependent on its underlying cause. Cases which are caused by infection can be treated with antibiotics. Other causes, such as kidney stones which have not passed, might require surgery. The key point of treatment is to drain the kidneys as soon as possible to avoid permanent damage to the kidneys. Kidney stents can also be a viable option for managing hydronephrosis.

---

[3] National Kidney Foundation Inc. https://www.kidney.org/atoz/content/medullary-sponge-kidney#:~:text=MSK%20occurs%20when%20small%20cysts,is%20considered%20a%20rare%20disorder.

PH of Kidney Stones

Acidic VS Alkaline Stone formation

Acidity is measured on pH scale, which can range from zero to 14. Common values for urine pH are 6.0–7.5[4]. Certain stones form in alkaline urine, while others form in acidic urine. Determining your specific stone formation and properly balancing your PH levels may help you manage your symptoms.

Why does PH matter?

If your stones form in alkaline urine, and you are ingesting items that cause your body to become more alkaline, you may increase stone production.

For example, lemon juice is touted as the greatest natural remedy ever for preventing stone formation, but it can increase certain types of stones that are formed in an alkaline environment. This is why urologists need to understand what type of stones their patients create, so they do not increase stone formation by treating with "cookie cutter" medical advice.

Over 50% of MSK patients create calcium stones. Getting a urine PH test is essential to care for MSK

---

[4] UCSF HEALTH. University of California San Francisco. "Urine pH test." https://www.ucsfhealth.org/medical-tests/urine-ph-test#:~:text=Normal%20Results,measurements%20or%20test%20different%20samples.

because certain stones form in alkaline urine while others form in acidic urine.

Stones that form in alkaline urine:
Struvite (magnesium ammonium phosphate)
Calcium phosphate

Stones that form in acidic urine:
Uric acid
Cystine
Calcium oxalate

Patients who develop stones due to unbalanced PH levels may also find relief by eliminating foods such as tomato sauce, peppers and fruits such lemons, pineapple or kiwis. (*This is a patient perspective and an opinion; not to be used to replace or provide medical care.*)

Citric Acid

Citric acid? Isn't that just lemons? Well, it used to be, but unfortunately, most modern forms of citric acid are not made from lemons but are derived from mold. Citric acid used to be made from fruits such as lemons, but corporations found a cheaper short-cut by producing a GMO form. This is now the common practice in America.

Chemist Carl Wilhelm Scheele discovered that citric acid could be naturally created by crystallizing lemon juice. However, modern companies discovered certain strains of mold could be used to synthetically curate citric acid and cut costs significantly. Citric acid is arguably the most used preservative agent in the modern world.

What is concerning about commercially produced citric acid, it is source. The preservative, which is derived from aspergillus niger, a form of black mold is in just about every product in grocery stores.

This fake citric acid is made by manipulating sugars exposed to black mold and filtered using sulfuric acid, which is a genetically modified organism. GMO derived citric acid is a common ingredient, food additive, and preservative which can trigger allergic reactions in those who are sensitive to it.

Is it Safe?

The Food and Drug Administration (FDA) does not mandate that companies state whether the citric acid they used in products is derived from natural sources or synthetically created.

Currently, there are no scientific studies that evaluate the safety of mold-derived citric acid when consumed for an extended period of time. There have, however, been reports of sickness and allergic reactions to the additive. Citric acid intolerance is not the same as a citrus allergy. Citrus allergy sufferers react to substances specific to citrus fruits, but people with citric acid intolerance react only to GMO derived citric acid itself.

Citric acid intolerance is not a food allergy, it is a literal physical intolerance to the compound. Intolerances occur when the body lacks some chemical or enzyme necessary for it to properly digest a particular substance. For example, lactose intolerance which is caused by a genetic defect which makes the body unable to produce the enzyme, lactase. Sufferers of citric acid intolerance lack the ability to process it. There are blood tests available for food allergies, but since reactions to citric acid are not IgE-mediated, there is currently no blood test for citric acid intolerance.

The University of Illinois in Chicago, USA published research[5] that explored how commercially produced citric acid could play a role in contributing to serious diseases. An excerpt from this study stated the following alarming statement:

---

[5] "Potential role of the common food additive manufactured citric acid in eliciting significant inflammatory reactions contributing to serious disease states: A series of four case reports" Department of Surgery, University of Illinois at Chicago, USA https://www.ncbi.nlm.nih.gov/pmc/articles/PMC6097542/#__ffn_sectitle

"Aspergillus proteins or by-products from the manufacturing process may be inflammatory with repetitive exposure. We conclude that there is enough anecdotal data to support the need for thorough evaluation of the safety and risks associated with the ubiquitous use of the currently manufactured citric acid in our foods, beverages, and other ingested substances."

In layman's terms, some of the test subjects who had diagnosed allergic conditions reacted to the Aspergillus allergen, unlike the healthy subjects who also participated in the study. Which may suggest people who already struggle with chronic conditions may find benefit from avoiding citric acid if it exacerbates their symptoms.

Patient Perspective Note- As an MSK patient, I have seen a major decrease in my renal colic and interstitial cystitis symptoms since I eliminated citric acid from my diet. When I accidentally ingest something that contains citric acid, I can tell within hours that I have been exposed to it. The renal colic and the classic "MSK kidney ache" increases each time I am exposed to citric acid. For anyone suffering with unmanaged MSK, I highly recommend a trial of avoiding citric acid for at least 3 months to see if it makes a difference in your symptoms. This is not medical advice, just a patient's perspective on something that helped me personally.

Life with Medullary Sponge Kidney

Living with medullary sponge kidney is a challenge, but you can still live a great, fulfilling life despite it. This chapter will help you create a plan of action to live your best life!

Being a rare disease, the treatment for MSK can vary. Diagnostic tests such as urine PH and stone analysis can help sufferers discover what type of stones their body makes and why.

Making the right dietary changes necessary for your specific stone type can be beneficial in the management of this disease, in addition to drinking adequate amounts of water.

Pain management is typically a necessary intervention in the treatment of MSK. Kidney stones are severely painful, and most patients need some sort of pain relief. Medications such as antispasmodics, urinary analgesics and even narcotics can be prescribed to manage the agony of MSK. Pelvic floor therapy is also recommended.

No two people are the same and you should discuss all options with your urologist. Most patients require a combination of lifestyle changes, nutrition, medications and physical therapy to manage medullary sponge kidney.

5 "Must Do's" with MSK

1-Understand what types of stones you create. Get the proper testing so you can get the knowledge to fight! Have your stones analyzed and complete a 24-hour urine panel.

2-Keep a daily log of your diet, lifestyle and symptoms.

3-Find a good doctor.

4-Get a plan of action. (Medications, lifestyle changes, nutrition, stress relief, surgical options, physical therapy, supplements & alternative therapies.)

5-Practice self-care. Eat, sleep, hydrate and most importantly, do things you enjoy!

6- Have a good support system with loved ones, friends, and/or community connections such as a church, social club or online group that can support you.

Mental Health

Make Yourself a Priority

You have to become your own advocate. This is your life, your body and your disease. You have to do what is best for you, there is no shame in that. If someone shames you for that, that reveals their character and doesn't change yours. The people who truly care for you want you to be taken care of. They want you to practice self-care. They want you to be well. If someone is constantly tearing you down, that is going to directly impact your health. Do not allow someone to make you feel guilty for things you cannot control. You didn't ask to have a disease. You didn't do anything to cause it so why would you take ownership and feel guilty over it? Guilt is a useless emotion. You can't blame yourself for something you had no control over. Eliminate anyone in your life who is making you feel guilty over your own health. You are worth much more than that. You don't deserve to be treated that way. You've been through enough. Don't expose yourself to any more pain! Kidney stones are horrifically painful. They can bring a grown man to tears. Give yourself a break.

Be Your Own Friend

One of the most beneficial lessons you will ever learn is to become your own friend. Your inner voice needs to be a positive one. You wouldn't constantly berate someone else for their shortcomings, why do you do it to yourself?

The reality is, disease can take a lot of things, but it can never take who away you really are inside. Your true character is revealed when all else is gone.

Don't beat yourself up because you can't do the things you want to do because of your disease or pain. Be your own friend. Care for yourself. Think positive thoughts about yourself. Hating who you are isn't going to help you heal. It isn't going to change your situation for the better. It will only drag you into depression. Pain and illness are depressing enough, don't add self-hatred to the mix. You are still you inside, despite any disease!

Adopt a Good Mindset

Replacing every negative thought with a positive one is a way to retrain your mind to be friendly. It becomes so easy to focus on the bad parts of our lives. When we switch our focus, our world seems much brighter.

It is important to take care of yourself, have a good doctor, eat, sleep and hydrate properly to achieve the best quality of life possible with medullary sponge kidney.

You are worthy of self-care. You are worthy of a life with as little pain and discomfort as possible. Never believe you are a lost cause. This world is full of a thousand possibilities. There is always hope. You are not alone in this battle against your health. Please take care of yourself. I promise you that you are worth it. You may have Medullary Sponge Kidney, but it doesn't have you.

Advice for Caregivers

To compile accurate information for this book, I created a survey that was taken by medullary sponge kidney patients internationally. One of the questions asked was, "How can family members, friends and caregivers help support you with your battle with MSK?" Below are some of the anonymous responses.

- *"Understand when we are in pain that we may have to cancel plans, also educate themselves on the condition.*
- *Offer to assist with chores, childcare, rides to appointments.*
- *Educate themselves.*

- *Go to appts with me, get educated on disease, ask questions.*
- *Understand when I have to cancel plans.*
- *Understand pain is real and very exhausting. Help with household chores as needed.*
- *Just understanding that when you have plans they can change anytime. Could be having no pain to all of a sudden kidney pain or stone pain in the bladder can happen then you have to cancel because of pain.*
- *Just be understanding.*
- *Just trying helps.*
- *Be there to take up slack, encourage hydration.*
- *Realize that though I may look "ok" I am operating at a deficit and struggling to focus through pain, Grace is needed.*
- *Tell us often: you are not a burden, it's ok to have bad days, we love you even on the bad days. Do the things we can't physically do like care for others, our home and property. Listen to our endless complaints.*
- *Be compassionate and understanding and believe you when you say you're in a lot of pain.*
- *Be supportive and empathetic to my condition.*

- *Help with chores around the house that are sometimes difficult due to pain and fatigue. Help be supportive and help notice signs of infection.*
- *By being knowledgeable of the condition.*
- *Believe the pain and symptoms are real and not in our head.*
- *Understand the pain is real, and just be there for you.*
- *By understanding that although I appear to be fine, I am often in pain.*
- *Be understanding and compassionate. Help when needed.*
- *Be understanding. Accept that even though you can't "see" the illness, it exists and has a negative impact on me.*
- *Share with medical team how their loved one with MSK struggles on a daily basis to function daily.*
- *Be there - listen and allow me to be heard and believe me when I tell you what's going on with me. Support, validate, and empathize with my feelings. Help to advocate with doctors.*
- *Understanding msk better. Knowing I can't do everything a normal person does because of chronic pain.*
- *Understand we have symptoms daily and have learned to cope outwardly, but that*

doesn't mean the internal battle gets any less.

- *Help when in pain.*
- *Just listen, understand and sympathize.*
- *By understanding the daily pain and discomfort I experience and that I don't have to actively be passing a stone to be in pain! Also, non-obstructing stones are just as painful as obstructing stones! All of these myths need to be rectified within the medical community because it's false!*
- *Education. Understanding the level of physical and emotional pain associated with the disease.*
- *Be good listeners, just understanding my moods will change and unable to always do things.*
- *Understand your struggle, be patient when you are short tempered due to pain. Most the time it is my own head telling me I am a burden and feel like a whiner.*
- *Understand and believe my pain. Allow me to have rest days.*
- *Help with day-to-day stuff when the exhaustion and pain is severe.*
- *Believe us, Read up on MSK, Have compassion, It's not all in our head, the pain. Help us when we are having MSK problems.*
- *Give me a break and let me rest!*

- *Be understanding, help with taking care of family and house.*
- *Understanding the pain.*
- *I wish everyone would listen and understand the pain and suffering we deal with on a daily basis. This is a lot to deal with. I struggle with pain and depression because I feel like no one understands or cares!*
- *Understand that I'm going through pain constantly, even though they can't see it.*
- *Learn more about the randomness of feeling sick.*
- *Just be with me when I am struggling. I don't want to be alone in my room cut off from everyone else.*
- *By being understanding and sometimes helping me physically with life*
- *Allow me to rest and recover guilt free.*
- *Get educated, understand crabbiness, believe my pain.*
- *Believe me, allow me to rest.*
- *Understand that I need to be left alone at times."*

As you can see, the responses indicated MSK patients want to be supported, understood and advocated for. Life with medullary sponge kidney can feel unfair and extremely daunting and having a good support system can help lessen the struggle.

Ways to Support

Encourage Rest.

Do not suggest your loved one "push" through their exhaustion. Respect their limitations. Be understanding that they are not lazy, and this disease can cause low energy levels. There is a reason the prefix of restoration is rest. The body, mind and spirit all need rest to heal.
When someone is faced with pain, surgeries, depression, and all the negative things that come along with chronic illness, it is important that they allow their bodies to restore themselves as much as possible. Naps, sleeping an appropriate amount of hours at night and resting on bad days are essential to living your best life with medullary sponge kidney. Encourage your loved one that rest is not being lazy, it is being loving to yourself.

Offer a Helping Hand.

Most healthy people will never understand the toll it takes on a chronic illness warrior just to accomplish "normal tasks." Everything takes energy! Showering, putting clothes on, feeding yourself, digesting food, having conversations, leaving the house, cleaning, doing laundry, etc. all take energy. I have found that people are quick to say, "I'm sorry you have this disease, I'll pray for you" but will rarely "Put feet on their prayers."

Additionally, very few people feel comfortable enough asking something like, "Can you come help me do a load of laundry?" or "Can you help me load my dishwasher?" One of the greatest gifts you can give someone battling with a chronic illness is your help. Often, just surviving takes all our strength and we look around at our piles of laundry, dusty shelves and sink full of dishes in despair; hating ourselves for our shortcomings. The truth is, no man is an island. We all need help at certain points in life and there is no shame in asking for it or giving it to someone in need. The old-world ways were very different than American culture now. Catchphrases like, "Fake it til you make it" resound in our culture. Which is terrible advice! Masking symptoms, pushing through pain and forcing ourselves into pure exhaustion and misery is not the way we are intended to live. Peace, harmony support and love were the resounding messages of the old world. Offer to help with chores. Volunteer to sit with someone who is in pain. Make them a meal. Mail them a card. Call them. Text them. These little things make a huge impact on someone who is struggling.

Advocate for their Care.

Medical post-traumatic stress disorder is a real phenomenon that happens to people who have a chronic illness. Many us have been gaslit, neglected and even abused in the medical system. This is why caregivers are essential advocates for their loved ones.

The pandemic created many issues for chronic illness warriors because patients were sent into medical situations alone. This was inhuman and arguably illegal. Should you ever be told you cannot accompany a loved one in a medical situation, use the information below to help you be by their side, even during a pandemic.

In the United States, there are legal mandates that state medical centers must follow existing guidelines in the Americans with Disabilities Act (ADA)[6], Section 504 of the Rehabilitation Act [7](RA), and Section 1557 of the Patient Protection and Affordable Care Act (ACA)[8]. North Carolina also passed legislation that mandates disabled patients have rights to have a caregiver with them during medical procedures, treatments, doctor appointments and surgeries, even during a

[6] Americans with Disabilities Act (ADA) U.S. Department of Justice Civil Rights Division https://www.ada.gov/
[7] Section 504 of the Rehabilitation Act of 1973
Office of the Assistant Secretary for Administration & Management. https://www.dol.gov/agencies/oasam/centers-offices/civil-rights-center/statutes/section-504-rehabilitation-act-of-1973

[8] Section 1557 of the Patient Protection and Affordable Care Act
US Department of Health and Human Services, https://www.hhs.gov/civil-rights/for-individuals/section-1557/index.html

pandemic, as stated in the SB 730: No Patient Left Alone Act. The Americans with Disabilities Act (ADA) states in Titles II and III that health care facilities are mandated to provide reasonable accommodations for persons with disabilities. These accommodations include the presence of a caregiver/patient advocate during medical events who can provide the patient with necessary support services, including communication with healthcare providers, support managing mental or physical health and other unique medical needs such as assistance with medical devices. Legally, no medical facility can deny a disabled person's right to a caregiver/patient advocate present, even during the covid pandemic. Standard legislation that mandates medical centers must follow existing guidelines in Title III of the Americans with Disabilities Act (ADA), Section 504 of the Rehabilitation Act (RA), and Section1557 of the Patient Protection and Affordable Care Act (ACA). These mandates allow chronically ill patients to have a caregiver with them during medical procedures, treatments and surgeries, even during a pandemic. Many pandemic restrictions crossed moral grounds. Patients with continuous ongoing treatments such as dialysis, chemotherapy and IV infused medications were forced to be alone during these already difficult treatment sessions Additionally, family members of patients in long term care facilities were denied visitation privileges, citing covid exposure risk as the reason why. This increased suffering and added negative mental health implications, which adversely impacted overall wellbeing to both patients and their loved ones. The increased potential for patient endangerment and medical errors in patients with rare disease protocols without caregivers and advocates present, should be of great concern not only to patients and caregivers, but to medical professionals as well. Facilities, hospitals and treatment centers cited covid exposure as the rationalization behind restricting visitor access and were not complying with the requirements of the Americans with Disabilities Act (ADA) which clearly states in Titles II and III that health care facilities are mandated to provide reasonable accommodations for persons with disabilities. These accommodations include visitors who provide the patient with necessary support. There are several federal disability civil rights laws that can apply to hospitals – Title III of the Americans with Disabilities Act (ADA), Section 504 of the Rehabilitation Act (RA), and Section 1557 of the Patient Protection and Affordable Care Act (ACA). All these statutes protect people with disabilities, and yet facilities, medical centers and hospitals across the nation denied chronically ill patients their basic human rights of support and comfort of a loved one during medical experiences. The ADA, RA, and ACA are not suspended during pandemics. Medical facilities must keep in mind their obligations under laws and regulations that prohibit discrimination on the basis of disability and that the federal disability rights laws remain in effect even during a pandemic.

Another noteworthy piece of information caregivers need to know is how to advocate in a medical setting for your loved one. In a hospital, one of the most important contacts is the ombudsman. A hospital ombudsmen investigates patient complaints and acts as a mediator between the patient and hospital system. Their entire job is to investigate and handle issues reported with the care offered by the medical staff and administration. The ombudsman is independent and impartial when examining and investigating complaints. If your loved one has been mistreated or faced a situation where maladministration involving negligence or carelessness occurred, do not hesitate to contact the ombudsman. Be sure you have documented the entire situation, have the names of the staff members involved and are able to communicate clearly what happened. It is also a good idea to get written testimonies from anyone who witnessed the event.

Be With Them.

Reminding your loved one that they are not a burden, they simply have a burden is key to supporting them. Battling a chronic illness is not only difficult physically, but mentally as well. If you sense your loved one is falling into depression, it is important to validate that their experience is difficult. Encourage them that they have successfully overcome 100% of their previous hard days and they have good days ahead of them. Let them know you love them on both the good days and the bad days. Remind them of their strengths when they feel weak. On bad days, they may not have the ability to go out and do enjoyable things. These are the days when the mental battle is the hardest. They may feel useless or even trapped by their circumstances. On those days, it is most important to just be with them. Your presence as they rest and recover can be an extreme comfort. In life, we cannot always save someone from suffering, but we can sit with them and help encourage them during the battle. Don't push them to do things they may not feel physically able to do. Gently encourage them to keep fighting and remind them better days are ahead. Understand that chronic disease can affect physical abilities, appearance, weight, careers, mental health, finances, relationships and self-esteem. Be kind, be supportive and understanding with your loved one. Accept them for who they are now and help them deal with the changes caused by disease.

Hope Healing Happy Clinic's MSK Protocol

Author of this book, Winslow E. Dixon, was diagnosed with Medullary Sponge Kidney at the age of 24; though she began suffering debilitating symptoms of chronic kidney stones, renal colic and frequent UTI's at the young age of 15. Her struggle with undiagnosed MSK caused her to develop another life-threatening disease, adrenal insufficiency, which almost took her life after a near fatal adrenal crisis on her 23rd birthday.

After being diagnosed with adrenal insufficiency, Winslow's health declined, and she discovered the treatment protocols for this condition had not changed since the 1940's. In order to save her own life and advocate for others like her, she established the organization, Adrenal Alternatives Foundation where she worked with stress-related conditions, adrenal diseases and cortisol care. Her nonprofit partnered with EveryLife foundation's community congress program and became a part of the United States Rare Disease Congressional Caucus to advocate for better treatment options. In 2017, the Right to Try Act was passed, which allowed for lifesaving treatments which were not, yet FDA approved to be administered legally under a licensed medical professional if the treatment was deemed effective and necessary. Her organization then worked to ensure lifesaving options such as the cortisol pump were available to adrenal disease patients. Though her professional work was a success, her health was still a massive struggle with both the medullary sponge kidney and adrenal insufficiency. To make matters worse, she was forced to make the difficult decision to have a hysterectomy at age 25 due to uterine fibroids and severe endometriosis. She also had repeated stent surgeries and fought to keep the chronic kidney stone formation managed. The repeated surgeries and chronic pain left her in a constant state of near adrenal crisis. Determined to get better, she began to research, learn and seek out any options she could to improve her quality of life. She continued her education and studied alternative healthcare, nutrition and natural medicine. Through what she learned, she slowly reduced the number of stones and began to stabilize with her cortisol. To her surprise, her alternative modalities that helped her regain her quality of life were regarded as pseudoscience and placebo effect within the endocrine community. A situation arose where she was falsely accused by another adrenal organization of dangerously promoting herbal medicine over proper endocrine care, resulting in her and Adrenal Alternatives Foundation being barred from attending a national adrenal disease conference. She quickly realized the stigma and limitations western medicine had regarding integrating holistic health into chronic illness care. Her credentials were seen as a danger instead of a positive in the western endocrine world, so Winslow made the decision to resign from Adrenal Alternatives Foundation and open her own naturopathic practice, Hope Healing Happy Clinic. Her clinic's protocols go further than your standard protocols in chronic illness care because they look into your lifestyle, genetics and stress levels. This chapter discusses her process for helping patients achieve optimal health despite having a disease.

Lifestyle Assessment: The goal of medullary sponge kidney disease management is to reduce stone formation, renal colic, flank pain and prevent urinary tract infections. To do so, it is important to find out what types of stones your body makes and understand your personal symptom triggers. We perform a detailed lifestyle assessment to understand not only HOW your body reacts but also figuring out WHAT it is reacting to and WHEN. We work alongside your urologist or nephrologist to compare your lab results to the lifestyle assessment, which allows us to have a deeper insight into why you may be struggling with quality of life, pain, energy levels, anxiety, depression, weight management and/or fatigue.

Define Your Chronotype: A person's chronotype is defined as their genetic internal master clock which defines circadian rhythm, regulates the sleep-wake cycle and other bodily functions like appetite and temperature. Depending on your specific genes, your body will function in a certain way and produce hormones according to your personal circadian rhythm modulation. Defining your chronotype will help you establish lifestyle changes and set a schedule that works best for your optimal health, energy levels and productivity. We work with patients to discover their personal genomics and create a plan of recovery tailored to their needs.

Food Support: Proper nutrition is not just about what you are eating, but when and how. We work with our patients to understand how to regulate their blood glucose levels and safely reduce oxalate consumption. Oxalates are natural compounds found in foods such as vegetables, fruits, nuts, and grains. They are also created in the human body as a waste product. In certain people, consuming oxalates may increase how much oxalate your body excretes in urine, which can cause the formation of kidney stones, increase inflammation, pain and cause chronic health physical and even mental health issues such as brain fog and anxiety. Our practitioners follow a low oxalate lifestyle themselves and have created a protocols to help you live and love your low oxalate life!

These protocols include:
- How to identify the content of foods. (Oxalate, sodium, nutritional content, etc)
- Calculating healthy ratios.
- Specific recommendations tailored to your body.
- Recipes.

Balancing Mental Health: Battling a chronic illness can present with mental health changes such as crying, anger, anxiety and depression. Panic attacks and an overall feeling of anxiety have been widely expressed by MSK patients. If you are experiencing any of these symptoms, please ensure you have adequate support. We offer counseling services both remotely and in person with one of our on staff ordained minsters to support emotional and mental wellbeing. We also offer biblical meditation which is a practice that combines breathing techniques, frequencies, meditation and scripture with an ordained minister, also offered remotely or in person to groups or individuals.

Complimentary Therapies: A noteworthy tool in the fight for health is the therapeutic use of alternative medicine and holistic modalities such as acupuncture and massage. Many alternative remedies can be greatly beneficial in supporting your health. However, they must be done carefully under the direction of licensed professionals, which is why we have a nurse practitioner and clinical herbalist on our staff who will review all medications and medical conditions to ensure none of them will interact with any natural protocols! Alternative medicine and herbalism are ways to support the body but will not replace certain medications. Never discontinue, reduce or change your medications without the advice of an overseeing medical professional.

Hope Healing Happy Clinic's Alternative Modalities:

Adrenal Health: Stress is one of the number one causes of mental and physical health symptoms and yet most people have never had the system that controls our body's stress response, the adrenal glands, evaluated. Our protocols evaluate how well your adrenals are handling the stressors in your life so you can improve your quality of life.

Biofeedback: The process of biofeedback technology is that it is able to tap into information about how your personal body system functions, in order to make adjustments to benefit your health and well-being. To evaluate a patient, our practitioner will connect you to small electrode pads (similar to a TENS unit) so the scanner can evaluate your body. Unhealthy cells or out of rhythm body systems can emit altered electromagnetic waves. Biofeedback technology can not only decipher out of rhythm frequencies but can also administer the right frequencies back into your body to support its ability to regulate itself.

Chromotherapy (Color Therapy):
Chromotherapy is based on the science of bioluminescence, which is the emission of light produced by all living organisms. The therapeutic use of color wavelength helps to promote balance and healing in the body. When the body is exposed to certain colors, these wavelengths emit energy and vibrations that either sedate or stimulate natural biochemical reactions such as hormone production. For example, in neonatal care units, babies with jaundice are exposed to blue light. This blue light exposure is used to break down an excess of bilirubin in the newborn's liver. (Not the same negative blue light which is emitted from cell phones and technology) Modern physicians also use light therapy in patients with Seasonal Affective Disorder (SAD) to help manage symptoms of depression and anxiety. Chromotherapists use specific colors to help promote healing by resetting the balance in the body.

Chronic Illness Management: Our intimate knowledge of alternative medicine, clinical herbalism and energy work helps us provide solutions to patients who may have been told by western medicine that there are no options for their care with chronic illness.

Cold Laser Therapy: During this treatment, different wavelengths and outputs of low-level red lights are applied directly to a targeted area. The body tissue then absorbs the light. The red and near-infrared light cause a reaction, and the damaged cells respond with a physiological reaction that promotes regeneration.

Tuning Fork Therapy: Tuning Fork Therapy offers physical, mental and emotional benefits. It is a natural treatment option with no known side effects. It reduces anxiety and promotes stress relief without the use of medication or other substances. It can clear negative energy from the biofield and aura, balance Chakras, and promote energetic alignment. This therapy can also provide physical symptom relief from issues such as headaches and muscle tension. It also supports the healthy movement of lymph, Qi, and blood throughout the body, making it a holistic approach to wellness.

EMF Protection: To reduce your risk of contracting health issues caused by EMF radiation, it is vital to learn to identify sources of harmful EMF exposure and discover how to protect yourself. We proudly offer a program that educates you on what can cause symptoms of electrosensitivity and gives you guidance on how to reduce your EMF exposure.

Holistic Homemaking: Learn how to identify which products in your home are potential health hazards and how you can replace them with safe, natural alternatives. We help you assess the products in your home and provide replacement recipes for items such as laundry detergent, cleaning supplies, make-up, shampoo, pet care recipes and more. You owe it to yourself to live the best life possible and take control of your toxic exposure and we are happy to teach you how! Consult includes a copy of the book, Holistic Homemaking.

Frequency Medicine: Frequency medicine is the use of electromagnetic resonances, tones, microcurrents and soundwaves to promote the body's natural healing abilities. Your body has a natural frequency that it resonates at. For example, your heart beats and produces a wavelength that can be measured by an EKG. Similarly, all organ systems produce their own frequency. When a cell or organ system becomes damaged, it can disrupt the healthy frequency. When these frequencies become out of balance, symptoms arise. An imbalance in frequency can cause physical, emotional and mental health symptoms.

Ultrasound machines can capture images inside the human body by sending sound waves into a person and collects the ones that bounce back then sends them to a computer to be converted into a physical image. Frequency machines work in a similar way by introducing the correct resonance back into the body. Introducing the body to specific frequencies is like translating the correct language to support an organ's optimal health. Frequency medicine introduces the correct tones to your body to help it self-regulate. Frequencies are simply translating a "language" the body understands. During the treatment, our practitioner will either use headphones for auditory frequency therapy or attach small probes, similar to a TENS unit machine to deliver physical frequencies into your body. The frequencies used during treatment are extremely mild — one millionth of an ampere. Such a small amount of electrical current is safe because the human body naturally produces its own current within each of your cells. It is a non-invasive, non-medicinal, highly targeted therapy. Frequency medicine is used to help the body enter a natural healing state. Precise frequencies can target the direct source and accelerate the body's natural recovery at the cellular level. They are used to reduce pain, inflammation and even emotional healing in a safe, natural way.

Though generally regarded as safe, there are certain groups of people who shouldn't receive Frequency Medicine treatment, including:

- People who have uncontrolled seizures or conditions such as epilepsy.
- People with implanted pumps or other medical devices.
- People with pacemakers.
- People with late-stage cancers.
- Pregnant women.

Frequency medicine is not intended to diagnose, treat or cure any condition and should only be used to support the body's natural ability to heal. Never start any treatment without first consulting your licensed healthcare provider.

Mcdullary Sponge Kidney Care
Medullary sponge kidney care is a fight you must take in stride with patience. In order to heal, you do not need to push harder. You just need to listen to your body and give it what it needs.
If you need MSK management, you can schedule a remote or in-person assessment at Hope Healing Happy Clinic!

To schedule your consult, book a timeslot on the website, Hopehealinghappy.com or call (941) 841-9903.

For more information follow our social media:
TikTok: hopehealinghappy_clinic
Instagram: hopehealinghappyclinic
Facebook.com/hopehealinghappyco
Youtube: youtube.com/@HopeHealingHappy

Medullary sponge kidney disease certainly presents itself with its own unique challenges, but it is not impossible to live a happy and fulfilling life despite this disease.

Proper self-care, medication and stress management are imperative to living the best life possible. My hope is that this book helped provide you with some information that helps you improve your quality of life. I wish you hope, healing and happiness.

Thanks for reading my book.

Sincerely,
Winslow E. Dixon

About the Author

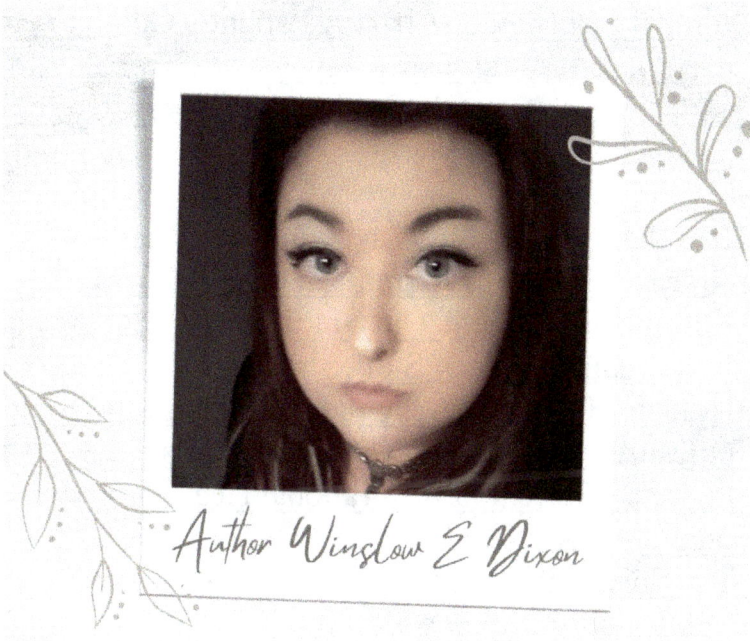

Author Winslow E Dixon

Winslow E. Dixon spent the last decade working with cortisol deficiency patients with the organization Adrenal Alternatives Foundation (now American Adrenal Association).

She helped to provide alternative care solutions to manage adrenal conditions and helped patients internationally to better manage their cortisol care.

For her work with the organization, she was nominated for the Rare Voice Award in 2020 by the Everylife Foundation.

Winslow has published multiple books on the topic of adrenal health including the best sellers, Adrenal Insufficiency 101: A Patient's Guide to Managing Adrenal Insufficiency and Cortisol Pump 101: A Patient's Guide to the Cortisol Pumping Method.

Her other published books include:
•Arsenal of Arrows Journal Challenge Series
•Chronically Stoned: The Guide to Winning the Battle against Kidney Stones and UTI's
•Holistic Homemaking: Guide to Identifying Toxic Exposure and Creating Natural Products.
•Peace by Piece 365 Inspirational Health Log Journal
•The Shivering Sunbeam. Children's book which explains disability in a way young minds can understand.
•Townsend: The EverVigilant Series, Fiction Adventure Series.

All are available through Amazon, Kindle E-book and Barnes and Noble.

In addition to her books, Winslow publishes articles on websites such as Yahoo News, Yahoo Lifestyle and The Mighty. Her poetry work has also been featured in many publications such as the Emerging American Writers Anthology and Florida's Emerging Poets.

Winslow lives by her mantra, "When you've been through hell, leave sparks of fire wherever you go." Her goal with her writing is to encourage everyone that even though your fairytales may have turned into nightmares, you can still slay dragons.

For more info on Author Winslow E. Dixon, visit her social media:

Winslow's Website- https://winslowedixon.com/
Winslow's Holistic Practice-
hopehealinghappy.com/
Facebook- .facebook.com/winslowedixon
Instagram- authorwedixon
Youtube- youtube.com/@winslowedixon

Sources

1. Gambaro, Giovanni & Goldfarb, David & Baccaro, Rocco & Hirsch, J. & Topilow, N. & D'Alonzo, S. & Gambassi, Giovanni & Ferraro, Pietro. (2018). Chronic pain in medullary sponge kidney: a rare and never described clinical presentation. Journal of Nephrology. 31. 10.1007/s40620-018-0480-8.

2. Tai-Seale, Ming et al. "Time allocation in primary care office visits." Health services research vol. 42,5 (2007): 1871-94. doi:10.1111/j.1475-6773.2006.00689.x

3. National Kidney Foundation Inc. https://www.kidney.org/atoz/content/medullary-sponge-kidney#:~:text=MSK%20occurs%20when%20small%20cysts,is%20considered%20a%20rare%20disorder.

4. UCSF HEALTH. University of California San Francisco. "Urine pH test." https://www.ucsfhealth.org/medical-tests/urine-ph-test#:~:text=Normal%20Results,measurements%20or%20test%20different%20samples.

5. Potential role of the common food additive manufactured citric acid in eliciting significant inflammatory reactions contributing to serious disease states: A series of four case reports. Department of Surgery, University of Illinois at Chicago, USA https://www.ncbi.nlm.nih.gov/pmc/articles/PMC6097542/#__ffn_sectitle

6. Americans with Disabilities Act (ADA) U.S. Department of Justice Civil Rights Division https://www.ada.gov/

7. Section 504 of the Rehabilitation Act of 1973. Office of the Assistant Secretary for Administration & Management. https://www.dol.gov/agencies/oasam/centers-offices/civil-rights-center/statutes/section-504-rehabilitation-act-of-1973

8. Section 1557 of the Patient Protection and Affordable Care Act. US Department of Health and Human Services, https://www.hhs.gov/civil-rights/for-individuals/section-1557/index.html

www.ingramcontent.com/pod-product-compliance
Lightning Source LLC
Chambersburg PA
CBHW071750270326
41928CB00013B/2867